Contents

What is Lupus?

To understand lupus, it is first important to talk about what lupus is. While this may seem like an obvious premise, in a nationwide poll conducted by the Lupus Foundation of America, only 39% of the 1,000 people polled knew what lupus was and 22% had never heard of the disease. This leaves more than half of the survey at a loss as to what lupus is. Of the people who claimed to know what lupus is, only 20% could correctly answer basic questions about the disease. While this is an unscientific poll, this sampling illustrates why there is quite a bit of confusing information about lupus circulating on the Internet.

The lack of information is partially because there isn't a lot of it. Researchers still don't know what exactly causes lupus or how to cure it. Lupus is also difficult to diagnose because it is similar to many other diseases. There also doesn't seem to be any reason for someone to contract the disease except for that it is nine times more likely to attack women than it is to attack men. So what exactly is lupus?

Lupus is a disease of the immune system, but in order to understand Lupus better, it is important to understand how a normal immune system works. The immune system is set up as a line of defense against foreign substances that attack the body like germs, viruses and bacteria that can cause the body harm. Even the simplest organisms have an immune system. Without an immune system, no organisms would be able to protect themselves against microscopic foreign invaders and they wouldn't be able to survive.

To protect an organism, the cells that make up an immune system must be able to differentiate between healthy cells, damaged cells that are sending out distress signals, and the foreign invaders that are attacking the cells of the organism that the immune system is protecting. With an immunodeficiency disease like HIV/Aids, the immune system is compromised to the point where it can no longer defend itself against invaders, thus making it predisposed to lethal infections.

The exact opposite is true with an autoimmune disease like lupus; where the super-strength immune system begins to attack both the foreign invaders as well as the healthy tissue, without being able to differentiate between the two. So instead of only attacking foreign substances that invade the body, antibodies and white blood cells begin attacking the organs and joints that have nothing wrong with them. These attacks lead to the initial inflammation and joint pain that is associated with Lupus, as well as the eventual scarring and destruction of vital organs that may occur.

To sum it up, lupus is a chronic, inflammatory autoimmune disease that causes cells of the immune system to attack normal and healthy tissue in the body. Whenever an immune system begins to attack the body it is supposed to protect because it cannot distinguish between the healthy cells and the invaders, this is usually the result of an autoimmune disease. Lupus is one of them and there are different types of lupus which can affect the joints, skin, kidneys, blood cells, brain, heart, and lungs.

There are other related autoimmune diseases, which include scleroderma, rheumatoid arthritis, and Sjögrens syndrome. Other diseases like diabetes and thyroid disease are also related to autoimmune conditions. Approximately

10% of patients with a form of lupus will also have symptoms of other connective tissue diseases, a condition which doctors refer to as "overlap syndrome" or "mixed connective tissue disease."

It is still not known why the body begins to attack itself in this manner, which is why lupus is difficult to diagnose and treat. In a lot of cases, it may take as many as three doctors and almost four years to diagnose a patient with lupus. Moreover, many patients have to go so far as to visit a rheumatologist (connective tissue specialist) before they receive their diagnosis.

Lupus is often referred to as one of the invisible diseases because symptoms may go into recession for years before it is diagnosed. As well, four out five patients continue to work after diagnosis without any obvious signs that they even have it. All of this makes it difficult to establish the amount of new cases per year as well as the number of deaths that are caused by lupus, its complications and related diseases. While the numbers of those infected with the disease seem to be increasing, it is difficult to determine whether there are more cases or whether there is more known about the disease that allows for more accurate diagnoses.

There is also no way to predict who will get lupus, although it seems to prevail in some groups more than others. Information from the Lupus Foundation of America indicates that somewhere around 1.5 to 2 million Americans have some form of the disease. Worldwide, there are 5 million documented cases of some form of lupus.

Amazingly though, ninety percent of the cases of lupus are diagnosed in women between the ages of 15 and

45. Even more remarkable is that lupus occurs two to three times more in women of color – including Blacks, Hispanics, Asians, Native Americans, Hawaiians and Alaskans. 70% of those affected with lupus suffer from systemic lupus. This is why that when most people talk about lupus, they are referring to this type, even though there are many other forms of lupus.

Lupus also doesn't necessarily run in families. Only 20% of people with siblings who have lupus will contract the disease and only 5% of children born to mothers with lupus will contract it as well.

Here are some more quick facts about Lupus:

- While lupus is predominating in women, anyone (including men) can get lupus at any age.
- No one knows what causes lupus.
- Lupus is chronic, even though symptoms might not always be present.
- Lupus is not contagious.
- Lupus is not related to Aids/HIV or cancer.
- Lupus is unpredictable and symptoms can come and go without warning.
- Most people with lupus can lead a full and normal life.

The History of Lupus
The discovery of lupus dates back to the Middle Ages, but it wasn't until the mid-1900's that any major breakthroughs were made. The term lupus (Latin for wolf) was coined by a thirteenth century physician Rogerius who

thought the facial lesions of the time resembled a wolf's bite. These are now known as discoid lupus skin lesions and were later diagnosed in the mid 1800's as a separate condition. Systemic lupus was diagnosed in the late 1800's when doctors began to put together the lesions with fatigue, inflammation, and other symptoms to form a more comprehensive finding.

Eventually, a combination of quinine and salicylates were used to treat the condition with some success. However, the concrete existence of lupus as a treatable disease wasn't established until 1904 by the work of two different doctors Osler and Jadassohn, respectively in Baltimore and Vienna. Finally, in the 1940's and 50's the disease was recognized as an autoimmune disease and lupus was able to be differentiated from other similar diseases and treated. Since the discovery of cortisone around the same time, patients with systemic lupus are now treated with corticosteroids among other medications. Currently, newer treatments are being sought to cure this chronic inflammatory disease with some success.

The Causes of Lupus

Because there no specific reasons for contracting lupus besides a slight possibility of inheriting the genes, doctors are only able to treat the symptoms and make suggestions to patients that they avoid situations that trigger flare-ups. There is an association of systemic lupus with the Epstein Barr virus, the virus from the Herpes family that causes mononucleosis, but that virus is present in 95% of people. As well, not much is known in the way of treating the Epstein Barr virus either, which leaves researchers at yet another dead end when it comes to treating lupus. Doctors have also considered the possibility that since lupus affects mainly women, hormones like estrogen may play a role in causing lupus, but have no proof of that.

So with regards to patients, doctors can only work with the probabilities of what environmental conditions may trigger lupus in someone who is predisposed to contracting the disease. These environmental factors include ultraviolet rays from the sun and also from some fluorescent lights. Patients are especially susceptible to lupus triggers and flare-ups if they take drugs for another ailment that causes sensitivity to the sun.

Other factors that trigger the onset of lupus include infections, colds, hormonal changes, exhaustion, injuries, emotional stress, and physical stress like a pregnancy. This likely assortment of triggers gives lupus patients many restrictions when it comes to living a life free of concern.

Because of the lack of answers with regards to the cause of lupus, there are many rumors about this disease. Most of these are unfounded and focus on modern developments like artificial sweeteners, silicone breast implants, and other recently invented chemicals that patients feel may cause this condition. It should also be taken into consideration that since it take so long to diagnose lupus, many sufferers have years to sit around and wonder what environmental developments are responsible for their illness. When the doctors have no answers about the cause, speculation is all that any patient has. This can start a patient on a frustrating and inconclusive search around the Internet looking for answers that simply don't exist.

Another reason why many rumors get started about lupus is because the symptoms can be so vague. These days, anyone can suffer from fatigue, low grade fevers, achy joints, chest pains, butterfly rash, and many other symptoms of lupus without actually having it. It is also easy for the media to blame lupus on many new developments in diet and other environmental factors because doctors have no evidence to refute their claims. If anything, all that doctors can do is say that it is possible that any environmental changes can trigger or cause lupus, which adds fuel to the fire that modern technology is responsible for many new illnesses that really have been around for a very long time.

There is however, one kind of lupus that has a specific and known cause. This condition is drug induced lupus. Drug induced lupus is lupus that is caused directly by taking drugs that include Procainamide, Hydralazine, Isonazid, Quinidine, and Phenytoin. Patients can reverse the effects of lupus by simply stopping to take the drugs. In the case of drug induced lupus, symptoms will fade after a few months. This is why medications are one of the factors that doctors will look at when they have diagnosed a patient with lupus.

Pregnancy and Lupus

While pregnancy has not been proven to cause lupus, it is associated with lupus due to the fact that doctors believe a change in hormones can trigger the disease. There is also quite a bit of recorded evidence that documents the likelihood of a lupus flare-up both before and after pregnancies as a woman's hormones change. A woman who already has lupus may safely become pregnant if she has had no flare-ups for six months before the pregnancy and is not on medication that causes birth defects.

Unfortunately, there will more of a chance of a miscarriage by a woman with lupus, especially in the second trimester when there is a danger of blood clot in the placenta. However, most women with lupus do carry the baby safely to full term. Women with lupus who are sexually active should consult a doctor about their contraceptive choices, as any birth control that causes a hormonal change may possibly have an effect on triggering lupus or lupus flare-ups.

Neonatal Lupus

Neonatal lupus is a temporary condition that may affect the baby of woman who has lupus. At birth, the baby may suffer from rare lupus-like symptoms that include skin rash, liver problems and low blood cell counts. However, these symptoms will disappear after a few months with no permanent complications. While there is a chance of heart defect, most problems with the baby can be detected during the pregnancy and can be treated before the birth.

The Signs & Symptoms of Lupus

The signs and symptoms can come and go over long periods of time and are similar to other many other illnesses. This is what makes Lupus so hard to diagnose. Symptoms may even flare up due to something like exposure to the sun during the summer and then disappear altogether for years. Symptoms also vary from case to case which makes lupus even harder to diagnose. So even people that suspect they may have something wrong may just go for a checkup and walk away with a prescription for pain reliever, antidepressants, and vitamins. Only 1 in for 4 patients with lupus qualifies for disability, so while the effects of lupus are devastating, they aren't always debilitating. After a while, all of this frustration leads some patients to give up on a proper diagnosis.

These are some of the more generic symptoms lupus patients suffer:

- Fatigue and fever
- Joint pain, stiffness and swelling
- Butterfly-shaped rash on the face
- Skin lesions that worsen with sun exposure
- Shortness of breath
- Chest pain
- Dry eyes
- Headaches, Confusion memory loss
- Purple or blue fingers when exposed to cold or during stressful situations
- Weakness
- Sores in the mouth
- Nausea, vomiting, coughing up blood
- Unusual loss of hair

As you can see, except for the butterfly shaped rashes on the face, there aren't many symptoms that distinguish lupus from many of the other ailments that it mimics. A person with lupus can have all or only a few of these symptoms. Since this means that no two cases of lupus are alike, it is important to look at how lupus is diagnosed.

Diagnosis of Lupus

Because lupus can lay dormant for many years and mimics many other diseases, it is difficult to diagnose. This is especially true because symptoms like fatigue and swollen joints can persist at moderate levels for years, being more of a nuisance than a warning. Some women may put off going to the doctor until they have the butterfly rash and even that can be misdiagnosed as psoriasis. At this point, even when lupus is detected, it will take several specialists including a rheumatologist to diagnose the disease.

Diagnosis for lupus is usually confirmed with an antinuclear antibody (ANA) test, but even this test can come back positive for perfectly healthy people. Antinuclear antibodies are what attack that structure of healthy cells inside the nucleus which contain the DNA. This is what brings about the damage in the body caused by lupus.

To perform the ANA test, a sample of blood is drawn from the patient and added to commercially prepared microscope slides that contain healthy cells. If the patient's blood contains antinuclear antibodies, then they will bind to the cells on the microscope slide. To observe the binding, a second antibody tagged with a florescent dye is introduced to the mixture. This second antibody will also attach to the already bound cells. Under a microscope, the original antinuclear antibodies will show up as fluorescent and confirm that they are present and attacking healthy cells.

Fluorescent cells indicate a positive test, while no fluorescent cells indicate a negative test. A positive test is then further analyzed to determine what sort of autoimmune condition the patient may have if any. However, about five percent of the population may receive a positive test with nothing wrong. As well, persons with viral infections, cancer, lung diseases, gastrointestinal diseases, hormonal diseases, specific blood diseases, skin diseases, and the elderly may receive positive results and still not have lupus.

So the ANA test is really only one part of the diagnostic process. Doctors will then go over clinical symptoms, medical history and perform other tests before making a diagnosis and starting treatment. Other tests will also be ordered which include a CBC, a chest x-ray, a kidney biopsy, and a urinalysis.

The CBC, or complete blood count, will measure information about the blood that the doctor can use to further diagnose the condition of lupus. The information includes:
  ➤ The total count of red blood cells (RBCs)
  ➤ The total count of white blood cells (WBCs)
  ➤ The total count of hemoglobin in the blood
  ➤ What fraction of the blood is composed of red blood cells (hematocrit)
  ➤ The platelet count

In addition, the CBC then provides further information about the measurements:
  ➤ Average size of the red blood cell (MCV)
  ➤ The amount of hemoglobin per red blood cell (MCH)
  ➤ The hemoglobin concentration per red blood cell (MCHC)

When these tests are completed, a patient must have at least 4 out of 11 of the symptoms of lupus, a positive ANA test and indicators form the other tests to be positively diagnosed with lupus. Once a patient is diagnosed with lupus and they realize it is chronic, they need to be aware of the long term effects.

The Effects of Systemic Lupus on the Body

Besides the symptoms, there is also the permanent damage that lupus will inflict on its victims including the damage from taking medications long term. Following, are the major organs that lupus will affect and how.

The Heart:

Lupus can cause the heart to become thick, swollen and weak. This can bring on conditions known as myocarditis and endocarditis. Lupus can also affect the tissue surrounding the heart, which is known as pericarditis which can be responsible for chest pains and shortness of breath. Heart disease is one of the main causes of death for lupus patients, so it should be taken very seriously.

The Blood:

Patients with lupus may experience different types of blood conditions which include leucopenia (a decrease in the number of white blood cells), anemia, or thrombocytopenia (a decrease of platelets which assist in clotting.) Diseases like leukemia and neutropenia are also common in patients with leukemia. Patients may develop an increased risk for blood clots as well.

The Blood vessels:

Blood vessel inflammation will be mild to severe, but it will affect circulation. Inflammation may cause small blood vessels to break and bleed inside the tissue causing them to appear as small red dots in the skin. Vasculitis may occur, causing many other symptoms like fever, feeling ill, poor appetite, weight loss, headache, blurry vision, seizures stroke, and behavioral disturbances. Hardening of the arteries may also occur.

The Lungs and Pulmonary System:
The condition of inflamed lungs caused by lupus is known as pleuritis and will result in breathing difficulties as well as chest pain when coughing, sneezing, or laughing. This condition can also result in fluid buildup in the lungs which can leak out. Pleurisy is a major concern because it is found in 40 to 60 percent of people with lupus. In some cases, patients may even develop pneumonitis which can also cause fever, chest pain, shortness of breath and a cough. Pneumonitis can be contracted from infections which may be a complication from medications that weaken the immune system. These conditions can also scar the lungs and make symptoms like a dry cough permanent.

The Gastrointestinal System:
The gastrointestinal system includes every organ from the esophagus down to the rectum and may be affected by inflamed organs due to lupus, and can also be affected from the medications that lupus patients need to take. Common gastrointestinal problems are acid reflux and ulcerative colitis.

The Liver:
An inflamed liver can also be the result of the medications taken to fight lupus. Jaundice, hepatic vasculitis, and autoimmune hepatitis are all conditions associated with lupus.

Kidneys:
While there is no pain involved, the inflammation of the kidneys caused by lupus (nephritis) will hinder the kidneys from getting rid of waste products and toxins efficiently. However, not all problems are caused by lupus nephritis. Patients with lupus may also experience kidney problems infections of the urinary tract, fluid retention, and

frequent urination that may be caused by the drugs used to treat lupus or other complications caused by systemic lupus.

The Muscuskeletal System:

Almost all people with lupus will experience muscle or bone weakness and pain at some point in their illness. This can either be caused by the lupus itself or as a side effect of the medications taken in order to fight lupus. Besides inflammation, some of the other conditions a lupus patient will suffer are lupus arthritis, lupus myositis, drug-induced muscle weakness, tendonitis and bursitis, carpal tunnel syndrome, osteoporosis, and avascular necrosis of the bone.

The Central Nervous System:

As lupus affects the central nervous system, patients may also experience changes in behavior, headaches, dizziness, vision problems and memory disturbances. More serious complications will include seizures or stroke. A neurologist may be needed to perform x-rays, brain scans, a spinal tap or perform behavioral and cognitive tests to determine what course of action should b taken to treat the problem.

The Eyes:

About 20% of people with lupus also experience problems in their eyes including changes in the skin around the eyelids, dry eyes, scleritis, sensitivity to light, nerve damage, and scarring.

The Skin:

A lupus rash or malar rash, commonly known as a butterfly rash, is probably one of the more devastating symptoms of lupus because it is a rash mainly on the face and can cause permanent scarring. This rash is mildly scaly and purplish or red in color and forms over the bridge of the nose and on the cheekbones in the shape of a butterfly, hence the name. The butterfly rash is not itchy, but can progress to other parts of the skin including the scalp.

The rash does not burn and is not otherwise painful, although it does feel hot to the touch and can become inflamed. Approximately 46-65% of lupus sufferers will experience the butterfly rash. Usually, in addition to the other doctors a lupus patient may have to see, a dermatologist is recommended for treatment in severe cases. During a flare-up, a malar rash can last for as long as a week and must be treated for quicker relief. Ultimately, suffers of lupus must live extremely healthy life styles in order to lessen symptoms like butterfly rashes.

Treatment of Lupus

The treatment of lupus will be tailor-made to suit each patient. This is because what each patient experiences with regards to lupus will be unique. However, no matter what course a patient and their doctors take, they will have will have to do it together as lupus is chronic and no natural way of healing will cover everything the lupus patient will have to endure and survive.

Because the ailments that are a result of lupus are so varied, there are many doctors that will be involved in treating this disease over the course of a patient's life span. Someone with mild or moderate lupus will see a rheumatologist who specializes in joint and muscle disease and can also treat related symptoms if they are minor. A patient with more serious lupus will have to see other doctors if they suffer from more serious complications due to more severe lupus.

For example, a patient with kidney problems will have to see a nephrologist. If they have the malar rash and develop scarring, they can go to a dermatologist. Other specialists like cardiologists for the heart, neurologists for the brain and nervous system, and perinatologists for high risk pregnancies may have to be consulted as needed. Having lupus can be expensive, costing about $12,000+ a year, with about one quarter of Americans with lupus receiving government assistance to pay their medical bills.

Lupus Natural Treatment

No one with lupus is recommended not to go to a doctor for lifetime treatment because with lupus, there is no way to survive the disease without long-term medical care. However, as patients learn to manage their disease, natural solutions become a big part of the treatment of lupus. In fact, natural solutions are especially helpful in treating and preventing lupus flare-ups and handling the symptoms of lupus without the side effects of long-term medications. Natural solutions mean that patients also don't have to go to the doctor as often for relief from mild pain and inflammation flare-ups.

Omega 3-Fatty Acids

Omega-3 fatty acids curb inflammation and help heal skin lesions, so getting a daily dose is an important for people with lupus. Omega-3 fatty acids can be found in oily fish, like salmon or sardines. It can also be found in flaxseeds and many other foods. Some foods even add omega 3's and are labeled as containing it as a supplement. If these foods are not available or not appealing, there are also omega-3 and fish oil supplements. Just make sure that they are from a reputable manufacturer and are stored properly on the shelves before you purchase them.

Other Supplements

There are many other supplements and herbs that you can buy as well. Just keep in mind that herbs and supplements may not be as effective because most of them haven't been evaluated by the Food and Drug Administration, but don't rule them out completely. Just make sure that you tell your doctor what you are taking because some herbs and supplements interfere with medication. For example, one herb not to take is Echinacea because it stimulates the immune system, which is something you don't want if you have lupus.

Ginger and turmeric are two herbs that are indicated as anti-inflammatory. Other herbs that have been studied are white willow bark, boswellia, devil's claw, bromelain, grape seed extract, reishi mushroom, pine bark extract, and curcumin. These herbs have been studied by researchers and have been found to relieve joint pain and inflammation in the neck, back and hip in many of the patients studied. These herbs generally replace aspirin and have been found in some cases to be easier on the stomach and more effective in long-term pain relief. Recommended doses are between 120mg and 240mg per day.

Food and Exercise

Since lupus is a chronic disease, diet plays an important role in keeping lupus as a manageable condition. More than anything, there are many foods to avoid if you have lupus. These foods can worsen lupus symptoms and help cause flare-ups.

Wheat and chocolate are two foods that cause flare ups. As well, lupus patients should avoid alfalfa, alfalfa seeds, and alfalfa sprouts. This is because alfalfa has an immune stimulating compound, L-canavanine, which also interferes with protein metabolism. Also avoid plants in the nightshade family – this means cutting out tomatoes, eggplant and peppers. Animal fats and omega six oils like sunflower oil, corn oil, and safflower oil should also be avoided. All of these oils promote inflammation. Lupus patients should also avoid high caloric foods.

While it may seem like lot to give up for the average person, lessening flare ups and keeping the disease under control naturally as much as possible should be the main goal for the lupus patient.

Exercise has also been proven to help patients with lupus. Studies have shown lupus patients who exercise can lessen their fatigue while strengthening muscles and improving cardiovascular fitness. While this may seem obvious, all physical improvements that assist in daily living help the patient with a better quality of life while researchers look for a cure.

Lupus Alternative Treatments

In addition to natural treatments, lupus patients can also find relief in alternative treatments as well. Whereas natural remedies are food and herb based, alternative treatments encompass alternative medicine. As always, a lupus patient should talk to their doctor to let them know what alternative treatments they are considering to see if these treatments conflict with any they are already receiving.

Most lupus patients do not rely on alternative medicine; rather it is used as a compliment to traditional treatments. The Natural Center for Complementary and Alternative Medicine, part of the National Institute of Health, is a recognized resource for patients of all types who want to explore alternative treatments in addition to their traditional course of medical therapy to treat lupus.

Reflexology is one treatment that many lupus sufferers have benefited from when it comes to fatigue and joint inflammation. Basic reflexology (a very gentle kind) can relax a patient and help them sleep better. This does improve overall health and well-being, in turn reducing symptom flare-ups. The most beneficial reflexology that a person can benefit from, with a possible reduction in medication however, is a more intense kind of reflexology. This kind of reflexology hits all of the points that directly stimulate the lungs, nervous system, heart, kidneys, liver, and other point of the body that are affected by lupus.

However, the reflexologist has to be careful not to stimulate the immune system because this will make a lupus patient very ill for several days. As well, stimulating the lungs, kidneys, liver, and other organs may stir up internal matter like mucus or other substances that have settled in various body cavities. This can make a patient slightly ill while the substances are eliminated from the body, but in the long run, may lessen the need for some medications.

Acupuncture has long been studied as an alternative healing method for lupus, but as yet, no conclusions have been drawn. A 2008 pilot study took a group of two patients to study the effects of acupuncture on lupus without drawing a conclusive determination. In the study, one group of patients was given medical acupuncture and the other group was given a "sham" acupuncture treatment with the needles being placed randomly. Both groups felt the same effects, which were both positive but not credible.

Acupuncture causes different results and different adverse effects for each individual patient. Adverse effects included bruising from the needles, lightheadedness during the procedure, slight fever, and transient bleeding. While there are many anecdotal accounts and many lupus patients use acupuncture, there are no studies or other proof that acupuncture is anything more than harmless or enjoyable for the patient.

Lupus Medical Treatments

Because lupus is a disease with many symptoms, there are many medications to take. There are other factors to consider when taking medication, in addition to the fact that lupus strikes everyone differently. Since lupus is chronic there are long term effects from some medications and also side effects, as well as other complications. This is why patients with lupus try to manage it with a combination of natural and medical courses of treatment. The most common medications to treat systemic lupus are anti-inflammatories, corticosteroids, antimalarials, anticoagulants, and immunosuppressives.

Anti-Inflammatories

Although anti-inflammatories are really just a fancy name for aspirin and other pain relievers, they are one of the most common over-the-counter medications that lupus patients take. This is because they work well on symptoms like fever, arthritis, and pleurisy; aspirin also thins the blood to help with blood clots. For some people with lupus, this is the only drug they need to take for their symptoms if they are mild. Aspirin and other anti-inflammatories can usually have someone with mild symptoms feeling better in about a week. The major side effect of aspirin is stomach irritation which may evolve into stomach ulcers with prolonged use. Acetaminophen is another pain reliever which is commonly used because it is easier on the stomach, but has no other properties that help with lupus.

Non-Steroidal Anti-Inflammatory Drugs (NSAIDs) like ibuprofen, naproxen and indomethacin work well because they are not only helpful with joint pain and stiffness but also suppress inflammation. All NSAIDs work differently, so if one doesn't work, a physician will recommend another to find the most effective one. Prolonged use of NSAIDs, other anti-inflammatories, can also cause stomach irritation as well as complications like bleeding ulcers. This is when treatment management becomes important. To reduce the risk of these complications, milk or antacids may be taken, or even additional medications like Misoprostol that prevent gastrointestinal complications. With both anti-inflammatories and NSAIDs, a patient should be careful not to take too much. This is why it is important to explore alternative pain relief and anti-inflammatory treatments if possible.

Corticosteroids

Corticosteroids are manmade drugs that mimic hormones which are naturally manufactured by the body like cortisol, which is made by the adrenal glands. Corticosteroids work like cortisol in the fact that they act as an anti-inflammatory hormone and also help regulate blood pressure and the immune system. They do this by lessening the immune systems response to attack healthy tissue and decrease the swelling, warmth, pain, and tenderness that accompanies inflammation of joints and other connective tissue.

Corticosteroids can be taken different ways, depending on the type of lupus suffered. They are usually taken by pill form, but corticosteroid topical creams are used for skin lupus and in more severe instances corticosteroids can be injected directly into joints or even skin lesions. The benefits of the shots are longer lasting, so corticosteroids may also be given this way to patients who cannot take the pills over an extended period of time.

Because of the side effects, most doctors give the lowest amount of corticosteroids as possible. The side effects include acne, hair growth, weight gain, and weight gain in odd places like the face, changing the appearance of the patient. Steroids also cause fluid retention and may cause the skin to bruise easily because it is more fragile. While the corticosteroids arc different from the steroids that weightlifters take, they still have some of the same effects. This includes growth suppression in children, insomnia, irritability, excitability, and agitation. These changes are associated with the higher doses, which is why doctors try to limit steroid doses as much as possible.

Since these steroids will be used for a life-time, there are additional long-term side effects that are of concern to the lupus patient. These include osteoporosis, cataracts, and drug-induced muscle weakness. Since steroids are only one of the possible drugs that may cause osteoporosis and avascular necrosis (destruction) of bone, lupus patients must take care to get the necessary nutrients to prevent premature bone density loss. Again, this is why many lupus sufferers turn to natural remedies and herbs to help keep them healthy. Long term use of steroids can also cause an increased risk of infection which is one of the leading causes of death for people with lupus. Keeping wounds clean is a number one priority for a person with lupus.

Antimalarials

Antimalarials work in conjunction with other lupus medications to reduce the dose of the other drugs needed. They do this by decreasing autoantibody production which also protects the skin against the ultraviolet rays that triggers skin lesions. Antimalarials also reduce joint pain, lessen skin rashes and mouth ulcers, and help reduce the risk of blood clotting. Antimalarials take much longer than steroids to work, but doctors prescribe them because the side effects are much milder than steroids.

The side effects of antimalarials include changes in skin color and upset stomach, but as the body adjusts to the medications, the symptoms go away. Large doses of antimalarials can cause damage to the retina of the eye. If this is the case, an ophthalmologist will need to be consulted. Antimalarials are also considered to be safe to take during pregnancy.

Immunosuppressives (Immune Modulators)

Immunosuppressives are stronger drugs that are used when steroids and other milder drugs fail. They perform the same functions of controlling inflammation cause by an overactive immune system, but because they are stronger, they have more side effects. This is why it is even more important to be monitored by a doctor if you take these drugs to control lupus. Infections are easy to get because your immune system will be greatly reduced, so any wound has to be monitored for redness, pain, swelling or tenderness. There is also an increased risk for developing cancer and liver damage when using immunosuppressives. If you need these kinds of drugs, make sure to find a physician who is experienced with them.

Anticoagulants, Immunosuppressives

Anticoagulants are used to thin the blood for lupus patients. This is because blood clots are another life threatening aspect of lupus and anticoagulants help keep the blood from clotting too easily. Again, regular doctor visits are necessary to watch that the blood does not get too thin. Also, since each patient reacts differently to the medication, they will receive a different dose.

Other Lupus Treatments

There are other new drugs which have been developed and even more drugs in different developmental stages, but other than this, there aren't any other known treatments (natural or otherwise) for lupus. The Lupus Foundation of America is very strict when it comes to recommending treatments both medical and alternative, and won't do it without the Food and Drug Administration's approval. Lupus patients are warned to stay away from alternative treatments that seem too good to be true and are not based on sound medical advice as alternative treatments have been known to worsen the condition of lupus rather than cure it. Because not enough is known about lupus, it is easy for patients to put out false hopes for cures that may be anecdotal and not actually helpful. In fact, because lupus is such a complex disease, anecdotal cures are known to do more harm than good.

Systemic Lupus

Systemic lupus, or basic lupus, is what most people are referring to when they talk about lupus. This is because 70% of people who suffer from lupus suffer from systemic lupus. Systemic lupus is the form of lupus that affects most areas of the body including the joints, lungs, heart, skin, kidneys, liver, and nervous system. Unfortunately, not enough is known about lupus to make it a preventable disease and it is also not curable. Rather, it is a disease that sufferers have to be taught to live with by learning how to manage their individual symptoms.

Systemic Lupus Symptoms

Systemic lupus is hard to diagnose because so many of its symptoms imitate other diseases. This is as hard on the doctors as it is on the patient. On one hand you have a patient who may insist that something is really wrong, and on the other hand you have a doctor who may be reluctant to diagnose lupus without absolute certainty because the treatments can be harsh and cause side effects that may make a misdiagnosed condition worse.

Systemic lupus has also been called the 'great imitator' because it mimics so many other diseases. This is why it may take several doctors and a long period of time to diagnose the disease in any patient. Also because each patient is different, each course of treatment will be individualized. Another reason why it is difficult to diagnose is because a patient may only suffer from a few symptoms, and these symptoms may come and go over time. Lupus is a disease with just as many remissions as flare ups. One thing about lupus that doctors do agree about is that there eleven basic symptoms, and a patient must have at least four to be considered a lupus patient.

The Eleven Definable Symptoms of Systemic Lupus:

Butterfly Rash

The butterfly rash is a persistent rash across the bridge of the nose that is the most easily recognized characteristic of systemic lupus. Only 30% of lupus patients get this, a condition that can also be due to rosacea.

Sunlight Triggered Rash

Exposure to sunlight will further worsen the butterfly rash and also triggers sores on other part of the body exposed to the sun, however this condition also has other explanations.

Mouth or Nasal Sores

These are pain-free sores that appear on the roof of the mouth and the inside of the nose.

Joint Swelling

Joints will not only be stiff and achy, but they will also be swollen and possibly red or warm, similar to arthritis. These symptoms will persist for six weeks at a time or longer.

Inflammation of the Lining of the Heart or Lung

This inflammation may cause a chest pain when taking a deep breath or when coughing and can also be due to a viral infection.

Urine Abnormalities

If the kidneys are inflamed and not working properly, proteins can be found in the urine along with microscopic blood cells. Urinary tract infections and kidney stones can cause the same effect.

Seizures or Psychosis

Since lupus attacks the nervous system, there may be nonspecific symptoms like headaches, but delusions and hallucinations are more likely indicators of lupus.

Anemia

The ANA test will help determine if a low blood count is due to an iron deficiency or menstrual cycle, or if red blood cells are actually being destroyed by the immune system.

Discoid Rash

This is a disc-shaped rash that appears on the face, scalp and neck that often leaves scars. This can mean skin lupus or systemic lupus and is a fairly common sign of the disease.

Positive ANA Test

Since 90 to 95% of the people who test positive on the ANA test don't have lupus, the test isn't conclusive on its own. This is because the test is actually used for many other diseases, which is why clinical symptoms have to be taken into consideration as well. The only thing that an ANA test can prove on its own is that if it comes back negative, you definitely don't have lupus.

Other Antibody Tests

For the person who tests positive on the ANA and exhibits ongoing symptoms of lupus, the doctor will perform more blood tests that will look for anti-double-stranded DNA and anti-Smith antibodies. These additional tests, along with clinical systems, will provide a definite answer.

The ANA test isn't enough and the clinical symptoms aren't either. While it is evident that these eleven signs may be experienced by a lupus patient, they may also be experienced in any combination by someone who has a completely different condition.

Conditions that exhibit some semblance of these symptoms along with a possible positive ANA test are: chronic non-viral hepatitis, primary billiary cirrhosis, drug-induced lupus, Sjögren syndrome, scleroderma, Raynaud's disease, arthritis, fibromyalgia, glomerulonephritis, chronic fatigue syndrome, and vasculitis.

These are less common diseases, but the following conditions and diseases are more common ailments that lead a patient to believe they may have systemic lupus:

- Alcoholism
- Asthma
- Congestive Heart Failure
- Dementia
- Food Poisoning
- Hypochondriasis
- Hypoparathyroidism
- Lyme Disease
- Pericarditis
- Pulmonary Edema
- Rheumatoid Arthritis
- Sexual Dysfunction
- Alzheimer's Disease
- Atherosclerosis
- Crohn's Disease
- Erythema
- Hyperparathyroidism
- Hypoglycemia
- Insomnia
- Myocardial Infarction
- Premenstrual Syndrome
- Reiter's Syndrome
- Rubella
- Tension Headache

Misdiagnoses of Systemic Lupus
It becomes obvious that when someone is in this kind of pain and that they think they have lupus, they are understandably inconsolable. However, the likelihood that someone may have arthritis accompanied by food poisoning and alcoholism is much more likely than lupus.

33

In fact, you can take any four symptoms from the list of the eleven lupus symptoms doctors use and chances are, at one point anyone will have experienced them together.

Especially if you look at symptoms like depression, skin rashes, fatigue, joint pain and other general symptoms, it is easy to see why someone may be insistent that they receive the battery of tests necessary to prove lupus. A doctor will however, be reluctant to diagnose lupus right away. This is out of fear of not only diagnosing the wrong disease and administering the wrong and harmful medications, but also from fear of ignoring what the patient's real problem is.

Because women are ninety percent of the patients with lupus, there are many more women's conditions that make diagnosing lupus an even longer process. This is why female patients that suspect they have lupus have to be very proactive when it comes to finding out what is really going on with their health. Internet research can be helpful, but only information from the Lupus Foundation of America is trustworthy. It is a foundation started by patients which is also open to alternative medicine, so it is a great resource for women to go to if they think they have lupus.

Another important thing to do as a woman is to look at all possibilities before settling on lupus. This includes diet, exercise, weight, alcohol consumption, birth control, age, medical history, mental history, etc. You will get a lot further with a doctor if you are honest about the information and have it summarized for your doctor.

Systemic Lupus Treatment

Unfortunately, systemic lupus is a chronic disease with no cure, and medication plus a doctor's care are necessary to lead a fairly normal life. While there are natural substitutions that may alleviate some symptoms, patients with systemic lupus will need to take some serious medications long term:

Prednisone Oral:

Prednisone oral is a corticosteroid which decreases the power of the body's immune system and in turn reduces symptoms like the swelling of joints. The side effects of Prednisone are nausea, vomiting, heartburn, loss of appetite, increased sweating, acne, and trouble sleeping. Other, more serious side effects may occur but are rare.

Plaquenil Oral:

Plaquenil (hydroxychloroquine) works to treat systemic lupus when other medicines fail by reducing skin problems and joint swelling. Primarily used to treat malaria form mosquito bite infections, doctors aren't quite sure how it works the way it does to treat systemic lupus. Side effects include nausea, stomach cramps, diarrhea, dizziness, and headache. Other, more serious side effects may occur but are rare.

Methotrexate (Anti-Rheumatic) Oral:

Methotrexate suppresses the immune system and interferes with cell growth to reduce joint damage and also helps with skin problems. It is a very potent medicine and rarely has been known to be fatal and cause birth defects. Side effects include stomach pain, drowsiness and dizziness.

Imuran Oral:

Imuran is an immunosuppressant that weakens the immune system and helps with joint damage by preserving joint function. This is another drug that is used when patients do not respond to more mild prescriptions. In rare cases it can cause blood disorders and cancer and the side effects are nausea, vomiting, diarrhea, or loss of appetite. Other, more serious side effects may occur but are rare.

Methylprednisone Oral:

Methylprednisone decreases the immune system's response to disease and in turn lessens swelling and pain throughout the body. The side effects are headache, dizziness, nausea, vomiting, trouble sleeping, heartburn, appetite changes, increased sweating, and acne. Other, more serious side effects may occur but are rare.

Kenalog Inj:

Kenalog Inj is a corticosteroid hormone that works by reducing the body's immune response and in turn reducing swelling while also lessening the effects of systemic lupus on the skin. It is given by injection and may produce pain or redness at the site of injection, weight gain, menstrual period changes, trouble sleeping, headache, dizziness, and stomach upset. Other, more serious side effects may occur but are rare.

There are many, many more drugs on the market to help treat systemic lupus. Most of these drugs including the ones listed here are in fact designed to treat other diseases but happen to work on systemic lupus as well. Until recently, there haven't been any new drugs aimed at systemic lupus, but there has been a new drug, Benlysta, which was approved by the FDA in March 2011. Benlysta is the first drug invented specifically for systemic lupus in about 50 years.

It will be some time before Benlysta is available for general prescription, but this is the first drug for systemic lupus that targets certain immune cells in the body. Benlysta targets an immune cell known as the B cells. These are the cells intended to mark bacteria and viruses for destruction by other immune cells, but in the case of lupus, mark healthy cells for destruction as well. Benlysta interferes with a protein critical to B cell activity and halts its search-and-destroy activity with regards to healthy cells. More studies are needed before it can be given as a prescription, but it gives hope to patients and doctors for a disease that has had little major progress since the 1950's.

Discoid Lupus Disease

Discoid lupus disease is a form of lupus that only affects the skin. While discoid lupus and systemic lupus are exclusive of each other; about 10% of patients that have discoid lupus will go on to also contract full systemic lupus, while about 20% of patients with systemic lupus will develop discoid lupus lesions. Since discoid lupus is a skin disease, and there are very few symptoms to go on for diagnosis other than the lesions, so a biopsy is needed to confirm a discoid lupus diagnosis for certain.

Discoid lupus is similar to other kinds of lupus in the fact that it causes cells of the immune system to attack healthy cells and is also considered to be an autoimmune disease. In the case of discoid lupus, the attacking cells are believed to be T lymphocytes which are a type of white blood cell - as opposed to auto-antibodies which are responsible for many of the clinical symptoms of systemic lupus. Much like systemic lupus, doctors do not know what causes discoid lupus. What they do know is that discoid lupus tends to run in families and is more prevalent in women of African descent.

Discoid lupus flare-ups are easily triggered by exposure to ultraviolet rays from both the sun and fluorescent lighting, even more so than with systemic lupus. Some patients are sensitive to the point of being burned and having lesions aggravated by the sunlight that comes through glass. Patients with discoid lupus are advised to avoid the sun altogether or go outside in the early morning or late afternoon if they want to go outside at all. Sunscreen is always recommended when outside and tanning beds are discouraged as they will produce the same or worse reaction as the sun.

Discoid Lupus Symptoms

The symptoms of discoid lupus are all concerned with injuries to the skin - which are inflammation, discoloration, butterfly rash, and the recognizable discoid lesions. Discoid lesions are coin-shaped lesions that appear on areas of skin that are exposed to ultraviolet rays, but also can occur on the scalp as well. These lesions may also develop thick and scaly formations. These formations are classified as either hyperkeratotic or hypertrophic lesions depending upon the structure of the lesion and how it heals. These lesions are not related to the nonspecific skin lesions caused by systemic lupus. It needs to be kept in mind that discoid lupus is a specific skin condition and is not systemic lupus - nor does it turn into systemic lupus.

Discoid Lupus Rash

A discoid lupus rash is a rash that usually occurs on the face, scalp, neck, and chest. These rashes can be flaky, itchy and scaly. Over time, they can also become hardened. When the rashes are on the scalp, they can become inflamed and also bleed and lead to hair loss or alopecia. White rashes can also appear on the tongue along with sores in the mouth.

Discoid Lupus Treatment

Treatments for discoid lupus are not as intense as those medications used to treat systemic lupus. Topical steroids are probably the most common treatment. Injections of more serious medications are used for the stubborn lesions that don't respond to topical creams. Other oral medications like anti-malarial drugs, corticosteroids and medications for psoriasis may be used for more serious cases or for patients that look like they are developing systemic lupus.

The main recommendations for discoid lupus are to stay out of the sun and extremely cold or hot weather. It is advisable to avoid fluorescent lighting and wear long sleeves and pants whenever possible. It is also advisable to join a support group or seek psychiatric help because the skin lesions are very visible when they are flared up and can leave permanent scarring which can result in depression. Discoid lupus patients can also benefit from eating the same healthy diet and using natural remedies as those that help systemic lupus patients.

Lupus Erythematosus

Lupus erythematosus is the umbrella term that covers all of the different types of lupus including systemic, discoid, drug-induced, and neonatal. These are all autoimmune diseases that attack healthy tissue in the skin, joints, kidneys, blood cells, heart, and lungs, causing pain and inflammation in these areas. Erythematosus is the Greek word for inflammation and reddening of the skin. While systemic lupus is the most common and the most devastating lupus to contract, it is important to understand each kind of lupus separately.

This is important because it isn't accurate to just say that someone has lupus. Saying this conjures up all kinds of worries and wrong impressions that are in many cases unfounded. For example, the headlines in the news may read, "Movie Star Gets Lupus" when in fact, they may have discoid lupus, or just a positive ANA test with some lupus-like symptoms. In the case of lupus, it is very easy to get carried away with misinformation, so education is important. Following is some information about the different kinds of lupus.

Cutaneous Lupus Erythematosus

Cutaneous lupus erythematosus is a form of lupus that causes lupus specific skin lesions. It only affects the skin, and it is not to be confused with systemic lupus which affects the organs and the skin. A person may have both forms of cutaneous and systemic lupus at the same time, or one or the other; and systemic lupus may cause nonspecific lesions in the skin which are not associated with cutaneous lupus erythematosus. This can be confusing, which is why it is important to understand that lupus symptoms may not necessarily be lupus specific, but rather complications of lupus or administered medications in general.

There are three kinds of cutaneous lupus: chronic cutaneous lupus (CCLE), subacute cutaneous lupus (SCLE), and acute cutaneous lupus (ACLE). What is different about cutaneous lupus is that unlike systemic lupus, it only affects the skin and is therefore treated by a dermatologist and not a rheumatologist. This is because cutaneous lupus is mainly triggered by sunlight. Like discoid lupus, cutaneous lupus also mainly affects women between the age of 20 -50.

Chronic Cutaneous Lupus (CCLE):

Discoid lupus actually falls under the umbrella of CCLE and is one of the most common forms. CCLE produces coin shaped lesions that appear on the v of the neck, the face, the scalp, and the hands. Once the lesions are healed they may leave a variety of damage behind them. This includes dark and light pigmentations, hair loss on the scalp, and fatty tissue that forms into nodules called lupus profundus. They may also leave indented scars known as lipodystrophy. Long-standing lesions may also develop into skin cancer and lesions of the lip and mouth may become ulcers. This is why it is so important for CCLE patients to see a dermatologist and stay out of the sun.

Subacute Cutaneous Lupus

Subacute cutaneous lupus is a lesser form of skin lupus and comes in two forms: papulosquamous lesions and annular lesions. Papulosquamous lesions are red scaly patches and annular lesions are ring-shaped with some scaling on the outer edges. These lesions can appear on the back and arms as well as the face and neck, but do not itch. These lesions may be accompanied by joint diseases but are not associated with systemic lupus.

Acute Cutaneous Lupus

Acute cutaneous lupus often accompanies systemic lupus. This situation is where the common butterfly rash is seen the most and looks like a sunburn. In this case the "sunburn" may appear in patches all over the body and are very sensitive to sunlight. These rashes do not generally leave scarring, but rather skin discoloration as they heal. As well ACLE along with systemic lupus can be associated with oral ulcers, hives and temporary hair loss.

Systemic Lupus Erythematosus

Systemic lupus erythematosus, the most referred to form of lupus when talking about the disease, is a misnomer in the fact that while it is the most talked about form of lupus; it is only one of the four different kinds of lupus in existence. Systemic lupus is the form of the autoimmune disease that affects all parts of the body including the heart, lungs, skin, joints, kidneys, nervous system, and liver. The most common medications to treat systemic lupus are anti-inflammatories, corticosteroids, antimalarials, anticoagulants, and immunosuppressives. However, these drugs may present further complications from side effects of their own, especially with long term use.

Chilblain Lupus Erythematosus

Chilblain lupus erythematosus is a type of subacute discoid lupus that causes purplish blue and red skin lesions in the form of nodules and rashes mainly on the fingers and toes and other peripheral parts of the body. This can also include the nose, ears, calves, and heels. In about half of the cases of chilblain lupus, these lesions will occur along with discoid lesions. As well, about 20% of patients with chilblain lupus will develop systemic lupus. Chilblain lesions are treated in the same manner as discoid or cutaneous lupus lesions.

In recent years, chilblain lupus has been reported to run in families, with childhood cases reported in more families than other kinds of lupus. Drug related chilblain lupus has also been reported and is associated with the diuretic drug hydrochlorothiazide, drugs of the calcium blocker class and by the anti-fungal drug terbinafine.

It should be noted that other medical chilblains (perniosis) conditions are localized inflammatory vascular lesions associated with prolonged exposure to heat, cold or smoking and should not be confused with chilblain lupus lesions.

Tumid Lupus Erythematosus

Tumid lupus erythematosus is a variety of chronic cutaneous lupus erythematosus. It is characterized by itchy red inflamed patches of skin which may contain extra moisture. The good news about these lesions is that they do not scar or cause the skin's pigmentation to permanently discolor. This is the main difference between tumid lupus erythematosus and other form of lupus that affect the skin. Tumid lupus erythematosus is sensitive to the sun and other ultraviolet rays and usually occurs on the trunk or torso of the body.

Tumid lupus erythematosus can occur in conjunction with systemic lupus or discoid lupus, but not necessarily. This is what makes it hard to diagnose, especially if it occurs on its own. Once it is detected, tumid lupus erythematosus responds to the same treatments as discoid lupus. An alternate name for tumid lupus erythematosus is lupus erythematosus tumidus.

Lupus Nephritis

Lupus nephritis is the technical term for when the kidney becomes inflamed due to systemic lupus. There are five classes of this disease, class five being the most serious. Class five only applies to 10% of patients. While most patients will respond to corticosteroids or other forms of medication, class five patients are likely to experience renal failure eventually. About one third of patients with systemic lupus will develop lupus nephritis.

Lupus Nephritis Symptoms
When discussing lupus nephritis symptoms, it is important to understand that not all kidneys problems that patients with systemic lupus experience are actually lupus nephritis. Kidney infections, fluid retention and loss of kidney function can be caused by medications like salicylates compounds and non-steroidal anti-inflammatory drugs. These complications will disappear as soon as the medication is stopped.

Symptoms that the patient will experience from lupus nephritis are swollen kidneys, urine abnormalities and reduction in the function of the kidney. There will also be side effects from the high doses of corticosteroids which will include:

- Increased appetite
- Fluid retention
- Weight gain
- Puffy face
- Easy bruising
- Moodiness
- Loss if minerals from the bones
- Cataracts

- Thinning hair
- An increased risk of infection and diabetes

Diagnosing actual lupus nephritis starts with the symptoms, but then requires tests to confirm it. Urinalysis is the most accurate way to determine whether a patient may have lupus nephritis. If a urinalysis reveals excess protein, red blood cells, or white blood cells; lupus nephritis may be a possibility and further analysis is required. A urine test will be conducted over a twenty four hour period to get a more accurate picture of the blood cells and proteins being lost.

Blood work is the next step to determine if the kidneys are working properly. A blood urea nitrogen study and a serum creatinine study will indicate whether waste products are building up in the blood. If protein is lost in the urine, a serum albumin study can determine the amount lost in the blood. Generally, with lupus nephritis, the protein levels in the blood will be low and further tests can measure if antibodies are high in the blood which also indicates lupus nephritis.

Once these tests have suggested lupus nephritis, a kidney biopsy will be performed. This is after an imaging study, which will determine the size and shape of the kidney. After a small sample of the kidney is removed using a small needle, the tissue sample is then examined under a microscope. This sample is then classified using the standards set forth by the World Health organization.

Lupus Nephritis Prognosis:

The prognosis for lupus nephritis is set by the <u>*World Health Organization*</u> *as follows:*

Class I - Normal
No evidence of lupus nephritis on the kidney biopsy

Class II – Mesangial Nephritis
Most mild form of lupus nephritis; typically responds completely to treatment with corticosteroids.

Class III – Focal Proliferative Nephritis
Very early stage of more advanced lupus nephritis; typically treated with high doses of corticosteroids, with excellent outcome.

Class IV – Diffuse Proliferative Nephritis
Advanced stage of lupus nephritis with definite risk of loss of kidney function; typically treated with high doses of corticosteroids combined with immunosuppressive drugs.

Class V – Lupus Membranous Nephropathy
Generally associated with excessive protein loss and edema; typically treated with high doses of corticosteroids, with or without immunosuppressive drugs.

Lupus Nephritis Treatment

In Class I and II, corticosteroids will be used initially. These are for the patients who have the most positive prognosis. Class III, Class IV and Class V patients will be treated with a combination of corticosteroids and immunosuppressives, of varying degrees of doses with Class V receiving the highest doses possible.

If a patient progresses through the treatments and eventually doesn't respond to the highest doses able to be given, the next step in treatment of lupus nephritis must be taken.

If both kidneys fail, this means dialysis and eventually a kidney transplant. In order to receive a transplant there must be no active signs of lupus while the procedure is scheduled to be performed. This type of transplant has been highly successful for many lupus nephritis patients.

Living with Lupus

Once a patient has been diagnosed with Lupus, they will be wondering how to live a normal life, when everything they have read makes it seem like that won't be possible. The fact is that there are many support groups, if not in the local area, then on the Internet. At this point, it is important that both the patient and their family and friends know that lupus is not contagious, very rarely hereditary and very rarely life threatening.

Exercise

Exercise is the first thing that a lupus patient is encouraged to do. Medication can weaken muscles and cause osteoporosis; lupus itself will usually cause muscle and joint stiffness. Exercising regularly can help prevent these symptoms and side effects from becoming more serious.

Fatigue

Fatigue from lupus is probably the hardest symptom to deal with, which is why a support group is necessary when a patient doesn't feel like exercising. Exercising is great for helping alleviate fatigue, along with stress and depression. Getting out with a support group is important for the patient. Staying inside and being alone at home only makes the physiological problems of lupus worse.

Rest

Lupus patients have to get their rest when they have flare-ups. This is why a good strategy is to plan ahead. Establishing set sleeping patterns, planning alternative and less taxing activities, and shopping and preparing meals in advance are all thing that a person with lupus can do so that if they have a flare-up they can still get the rest that they need without getting fatigued.

Sensitivity to Light

Since two-thirds of patients that suffer from lupus will be sensitive to ultraviolet light, sunscreen along with long sleeves and pants will have to be worn when out in the sun. The strongest hours of sunlight are between 10AM and 4PM, so be sure to avoid the sun during that time. Ultraviolet light is also given off by some fluorescent lighting, but there are shields for that can be purchased to cover them. Not being out in the sun may be difficult on some patients, but it simply cannot be helped. Tanning beds are also not safe for patients with lupus.

Conclusion - Hope for the Future

Ongoing research is currently being conducted in independent studies to discover a cure for lupus, focusing on families that have more than one member who has lupus to discover some hereditary link. The Lupus Foundation of America is perhaps the largest research support group, and also has many answers for this unexplained disease, but no real cure in the near future.

In a survey conducted by the LFA, they found that out of those with lupus who responded 78% said they were coping well with lupus and that 72% said family and friends were supportive. 84% said that family members were there primary support network and 72% said it was their friends as well. As far as the difficulty of living with lupus - the pain of lupus, lifestyle changes, and emotional problems ranked as the three most difficult problems to cope with, in that order.

However, while lupus may be a chronic disease, it is not a fatal one. Only one in four cases of diagnosed lupus patients collect disability in the United States and there are many success stories of people that don't let lupus get them down, no matter what they have to endure to get through the day. Lupus is a manageable disease with breakthroughs to come and lots of worldwide support. So a diagnosis of lupus does not mean a prognosis that has to be bleak, and living with lupus can still mean achieving life-long goals.